EMMANUEL JOSEPH

The Sacred Scaffold, A Journey Through Myth, Medicine, and Architectural Innovation

Copyright © 2025 by Emmanuel Joseph

All rights reserved. No part of this publication may be reproduced, stored or transmitted in any form or by any means, electronic, mechanical, photocopying, recording, scanning, or otherwise without written permission from the publisher. It is illegal to copy this book, post it to a website, or distribute it by any other means without permission.

First edition

This book was professionally typeset on Reedsy. Find out more at reedsy.com

Contents

1. Chapter 1: The Origin of Myths — 1
2. Chapter 2: Healing in the Hands of the Gods — 3
3. Chapter 3: The Alchemy of Architecture — 5
4. Chapter 4: Bridging Realms with Bridges — 7
5. Chapter 5: The Sacred Geometry of Cathedrals — 9
6. Chapter 6: Renaissance Revival — 11
7. Chapter 7: The Industrial Revolution and Urban Myths — 13
8. Chapter 8: Modern Medicine and Myth — 15
9. Chapter 9: Sustainable Architecture — 17
10. Chapter 10: The Digital Age and Virtual Realities — 19
11. Chapter 11: Rediscovering Ancient Wisdom — 21
12. Chapter 12: Building the Future — 23
13. Chapter 13: The Power of Symbols — 25
14. Chapter 14: The Healing Power of Nature — 27
15. Chapter 15: The Global Exchange of Knowledge — 29

1

Chapter 1: The Origin of Myths

In the beginning, humanity was in awe of the mysteries of the world around them. They gazed upon the stars, the mountains, and the oceans, crafting tales to explain their existence. Myths emerged from every culture, embodying the values, fears, and aspirations of ancient peoples. These stories were more than mere entertainment; they were the framework upon which societies built their understanding of life and the cosmos. From the creation myths of the Greeks to the ancestral legends of the African tribes, each tale provided a sacred scaffold, a structure that connected the mundane to the divine.

As these myths evolved, they began to shape the collective consciousness of societies. They were passed down through generations, serving as a means of preserving cultural identity and heritage. The oral tradition played a crucial role in this process, with storytellers becoming the custodians of ancient wisdom. These narratives were not static; they adapted to changing times and circumstances, reflecting the dynamic nature of human experience. Myths also served as moral guides, imparting lessons on virtues such as bravery, wisdom, and compassion.

In addition to their cultural significance, myths had a profound impact on early scientific thought. Ancient peoples sought to understand the natural world through the lens of their mythology. Phenomena such as eclipses, thunderstorms, and earthquakes were explained through the actions of gods and spirits. While these explanations may seem primitive by modern standards, they represented an important step in humanity's quest for knowledge. Myths laid the groundwork for the development of more sophisticated scientific theories and practices.

Furthermore, myths played a central role in the construction of sacred spaces. Temples, shrines, and other religious structures were often designed with mythological symbolism in mind. The placement of these buildings, their architectural features, and the rituals performed within them were all influenced by the stories that shaped the spiritual beliefs of the people. In this way, myths became the foundation upon which the physical and metaphysical aspects of society were built, creating a sacred scaffold that connected the human and the divine.

2

Chapter 2: Healing in the Hands of the Gods

As societies evolved, so did their understanding of health and disease. Ancient medicine was deeply intertwined with myth and religion. Shamans, priests, and healers were seen as intermediaries between the gods and humanity, possessing sacred knowledge that could cure ailments. The Egyptians revered Imhotep, a polymath who was later deified as the god of medicine. Similarly, in Greece, Asclepius was worshipped as a divine healer. These figures exemplified the belief that healing was a divine gift, and their practices laid the foundation for modern medicine.

In ancient Egypt, the practice of medicine was closely linked to religious beliefs. Temples dedicated to healing gods, such as Imhotep and Thoth, served as centers of medical knowledge and treatment. These temples were equipped with libraries containing medical texts, as well as facilities for surgery and other treatments. The priests who served in these temples were not only religious figures but also skilled physicians. They believed that illness was caused by supernatural forces and that healing required the intervention of the gods.

In Greece, the cult of Asclepius played a similar role in the development of medical practices. Asclepius was believed to possess the power to heal the sick and even raise the dead. Temples dedicated to him, known as Asclepieia, were established throughout the Greek world. These temples functioned as healing centers, where patients would undergo rituals and treatments designed to restore their health. The methods used in these temples were a blend of religious practices and empirical observations, laying the groundwork for the later development of scientific medicine.

The influence of these ancient traditions can still be seen in modern medicine. Many of the symbols and practices associated with contemporary healthcare have their roots in these ancient cultures. The caduceus, a staff entwined with serpents, is a symbol of medicine that dates back to the worship of Asclepius. The holistic approach to healing, which emphasizes the connection between mind, body, and spirit, can also be traced back to these early medical practices. By understanding the origins of these traditions, we can gain a deeper appreciation for the rich tapestry of knowledge that has shaped modern medicine.

3

Chapter 3: The Alchemy of Architecture

Architecture is not merely the creation of physical structures; it is the manifestation of cultural and spiritual values. Ancient builders infused their work with symbolic meanings, creating spaces that were not just functional but also sacred. The ziggurats of Mesopotamia, the pyramids of Egypt, and the temples of Greece were all designed to bridge the human and the divine. These monumental structures served as stages for rituals, reinforcing the sacred myths and medical knowledge of their time. Each stone, each column, was a testament to the ingenuity and reverence of the builders.

The construction of these ancient wonders required a profound understanding of both engineering and spirituality. Builders employed advanced techniques to achieve precise alignments and proportions, often using astronomical observations to guide their work. The pyramids of Egypt, for example, were aligned with the cardinal points and incorporated complex mathematical principles. These structures were not just tombs for pharaohs; they were believed to be gateways to the afterlife, connecting the earthly realm with the divine.

In Mesopotamia, the ziggurats were towering structures that served as temples and administrative centers. These stepped pyramids were designed to represent the cosmic mountain, a sacred axis that connected heaven and earth. The construction of ziggurats required the labor of thousands of workers and the expertise of skilled craftsmen. Their imposing presence dominated the landscape, symbolizing the power and authority of the gods and the rulers who built them.

The temples of Greece, with their elegant columns and intricate sculptures, were masterpieces of architectural innovation. The Greeks believed that the gods resided in these temples, and every aspect of their design was intended to honor the divine. The Parthenon, dedicated to the goddess Athena, is a prime example of this blend of artistry and spirituality. Its proportions were calculated to create a sense of harmony and balance, reflecting the Greek ideal of beauty. The sculptures that adorned the temple depicted scenes from mythology, reinforcing the sacred narratives that shaped Greek culture.

These ancient architectural marvels continue to inspire awe and admiration today. They stand as a testament to the creativity and dedication of the builders who constructed them, as well as the enduring power of the myths that inspired their creation. By studying these structures, we can gain insight into the cultural and spiritual values of ancient civilizations and appreciate the profound connection between architecture and the sacred.

4

Chapter 4: Bridging Realms with Bridges

Bridges have always been more than just means of crossing physical barriers; they symbolize the connection between different realms. In mythology, bridges often represented the passage from the mortal world to the divine. The Bifröst in Norse mythology connected Midgard (the world of humans) with Asgard (the realm of the gods). In reality, the construction of bridges was a significant architectural and engineering challenge. The Romans, with their mastery of the arch, revolutionized bridge-building, creating structures that stood the test of time and symbolized the enduring connection between different parts of the empire.

The importance of bridges in human history cannot be overstated. They facilitated trade, communication, and cultural exchange, helping to shape the development of civilizations. The bridges built by the Romans, such as the Pont du Gard in France, are remarkable examples of their engineering prowess. These structures were designed to withstand the forces of nature, using a combination of arches and durable materials. The ability to build such robust and enduring bridges enabled the Romans to expand their empire and maintain control over vast territories.

In medieval Europe, the construction of bridges took on a new dimension with the rise of the Gothic style. The use of pointed arches and ribbed vaults allowed for greater height and stability, enabling the creation of more elaborate and visually stunning structures. One of the most famous examples is the Charles Bridge in Prague, adorned with statues of saints and other religious figures. This bridge not only served as a vital crossing point over the Vltava River but also as a symbol of the city's spiritual and cultural identity.

The symbolic significance of bridges continues to resonate in modern times. Contemporary architects and engineers draw inspiration from the past while incorporating new materials and technologies. The Golden Gate Bridge in San Francisco, with its iconic red color and sweeping suspension cables, has become a symbol of innovation and resilience. As we move forward, the construction of bridges will continue to represent the enduring human desire to connect, transcend, and explore new horizons.

5

Chapter 5: The Sacred Geometry of Cathedrals

The cathedrals of medieval Europe are marvels of architectural innovation and spiritual expression. Their design was deeply influenced by sacred geometry, a belief that certain shapes and proportions had divine significance. The architects of these grand structures believed that by incorporating these principles, they were creating a space where the divine could reside. The soaring arches, the intricate stained glass windows, and the majestic spires all combined to create a sense of awe and reverence. These cathedrals were not just places of worship; they were physical manifestations of the sacred scaffold that connected humanity to the divine.

The use of sacred geometry in cathedral design can be seen in the meticulous planning and execution of their layouts. The proportions of these structures were often based on mathematical ratios, such as the Golden Ratio, which were believed to embody harmony and beauty. The floor plans of cathedrals, typically in the shape of a cross, were designed to reflect the Christian faith and its teachings. Each element, from the height of the nave to the placement of the altar, was carefully considered to create a space that inspired spiritual contemplation and devotion.

Stained glass windows played a crucial role in the spiritual experience of cathedral visitors. These windows depicted scenes from the Bible, saints, and other religious symbols, serving as visual sermons for the congregation. The use of vibrant colors and intricate designs transformed the light that entered the cathedral, creating a transcendent atmosphere. The craftsmanship involved in creating these windows was unparalleled, with artisans using techniques that have been passed down through generations.

The construction of cathedrals required the collaboration of skilled craftsmen, architects, and laborers. These projects often took decades, or even centuries, to complete. The dedication and artistry of those who built these structures are evident in every detail, from the delicate carvings to the towering spires. The legacy of these cathedrals extends beyond their architectural achievements; they stand as a testament to the human spirit's quest for connection with the divine and the creation of spaces that elevate the soul.

6

Chapter 6: Renaissance Revival

The Renaissance was a period of rediscovery and innovation. Inspired by the classical knowledge of Greece and Rome, architects, artists, and scientists sought to create a new era of enlightenment. The mythological and medical knowledge of the ancients was reinterpreted and integrated into the fabric of Renaissance society. The works of Leonardo da Vinci epitomize this synthesis. His studies of human anatomy, informed by ancient texts, led to advancements in medicine, while his architectural designs reflected the principles of harmony and proportion that were central to classical myths.

During the Renaissance, there was a renewed interest in the works of ancient philosophers and scholars. Texts that had been lost or forgotten were rediscovered, translated, and studied. This revival of classical knowledge had a profound impact on all areas of society, including medicine and architecture. Renaissance architects drew inspiration from the symmetry and proportions of ancient Roman and Greek structures, creating buildings that emphasized balance and beauty. The use of columns, arches, and domes became hallmarks of Renaissance architecture.

Leonardo da Vinci, one of the most celebrated figures of the Renaissance, exemplified the era's spirit of curiosity and innovation. His detailed anatomical studies, based on dissections of human bodies, provided invaluable insights into the structure and function of the human form. These studies not only advanced medical knowledge but also informed his artistic work. Leonardo's Vitruvian Man, a drawing that illustrates the ideal human proportions, is a perfect example of the intersection of art, science, and mythology that characterized the Renaissance.

The architectural achievements of the Renaissance were not limited to Italy. The movement spread throughout Europe, influencing the design of buildings in France, England, Spain, and beyond. The Château de Chambord in France, with its blend of medieval and classical elements, is a stunning example of Renaissance architecture. Similarly, St. Peter's Basilica in Vatican City, with its grand dome designed by Michelangelo, embodies the principles of Renaissance design and serves as a symbol of the Catholic Church's power and influence.

The Renaissance was a time of great cultural and intellectual growth. By looking back to the wisdom of the ancients and incorporating their knowledge into contemporary practices, Renaissance thinkers and creators laid the groundwork for many of the advancements that followed. Their work continues to inspire and inform modern medicine, architecture, and the arts, demonstrating the enduring power of the sacred scaffold that connects past and present.

7

Chapter 7: The Industrial Revolution and Urban Myths

The Industrial Revolution brought about a dramatic transformation in society and architecture. The rapid urbanization and technological advancements created a new set of myths and challenges. Skyscrapers, factories, and railways became the new symbols of progress. However, these innovations also brought about new myths, such as the fear of dehumanization and loss of individuality. Urban legends and tales of haunted factories emerged, reflecting the anxieties of a rapidly changing world. The architecture of this era, with its emphasis on functionality and efficiency, marked a departure from the sacred and mythical structures of the past.

The construction of skyscrapers during the Industrial Revolution represented a significant leap in architectural and engineering capabilities. These towering structures, made possible by advancements in steel production and elevator technology, became symbols of modernity and progress. The iconic skyline of New York City, with its early skyscrapers like the Flatiron Building and the Empire State Building, embodied the spirit of innovation and ambition. However, the rapid rise of urban environments also led to concerns about the impact on human well-being and the loss of connection to nature.

Factories, another hallmark of the Industrial Revolution, revolutionized the production process but also introduced new challenges. The shift from artisanal craftsmanship to mass production resulted in a loss of individuality and a sense of alienation among workers. Factory towns, with their uniform rows of worker housing and the imposing presence of industrial facilities, became the backdrop for new urban myths and legends. Stories of haunted factories and ghostly apparitions reflected the fears and uncertainties of a rapidly changing society.

Railways, which facilitated the movement of goods and people across vast distances, also played a crucial role in the transformation of the urban landscape. The construction of railway stations and bridges required innovative engineering solutions and contributed to the spread of architectural styles. The grand railway stations of the 19th century, such as St. Pancras in London and Grand Central Terminal in New York, combined functionality with aesthetic appeal, becoming iconic landmarks in their own right. These structures, while emblematic of progress, also evoked a sense of nostalgia for a bygone era.

The Industrial Revolution was a period of profound change that reshaped the built environment and gave rise to new myths and legends. The architectural innovations of this era laid the groundwork for the modern city, while the stories and anxieties that emerged from this transformation continue to influence contemporary culture. By examining the myths and architectural achievements of the Industrial Revolution, we gain a deeper understanding of the complex interplay between progress, technology, and the human experience.

8

Chapter 8: Modern Medicine and Myth

The 20th century witnessed unprecedented advancements in medicine. Discoveries in microbiology, genetics, and pharmacology transformed healthcare. Yet, even in this age of scientific progress, myths persisted. The placebo effect, for example, demonstrated the power of belief in the healing process. Modern medicine also grappled with ethical dilemmas, such as cloning and genetic modification, which evoked age-old questions about the nature of life and the role of humanity in altering it. These contemporary issues, while grounded in science, still resonated with the myths and moral questions that have been part of human history.

The discovery of antibiotics revolutionized the treatment of bacterial infections and saved countless lives. However, the overuse and misuse of these medications led to the emergence of antibiotic-resistant strains of bacteria, posing new challenges for healthcare providers. The development of vaccines, such as the polio vaccine, eradicated deadly diseases and highlighted the importance of preventive medicine. Despite these advancements, myths and misconceptions about vaccines persisted, leading to vaccine hesitancy and outbreaks of preventable diseases.

Genetic research and the mapping of the human genome opened new frontiers in medicine, enabling personalized treatments and the potential for gene therapy. However, these advancements also raised ethical questions about the manipulation of genetic material. The concept of "playing God" and altering the fundamental building blocks of life resonated with age-old myths about the consequences of hubris and the limits of human knowledge. Debates about the morality of cloning, genetic engineering, and designer babies continue to shape public discourse and policy.

The placebo effect, a phenomenon where patients experience improvements in their condition due to their belief in the treatment, underscores the complex relationship between mind and body in the healing process. This effect highlights the power of belief and the importance of considering psychological and emotional factors in medical treatment. The placebo effect also challenges the strictly mechanistic view of medicine, suggesting that healing involves more than just physical interventions.

Modern medicine has made remarkable strides in diagnosing, treating, and preventing diseases. However, it also faces ongoing challenges and ethical dilemmas that require a nuanced understanding of both scientific principles and the myths that shape human beliefs and behaviors. By examining the interplay between myth and medicine, we can better appreciate the complexities of healthcare and the importance of addressing both the physical and psychological aspects of healing.

9

Chapter 9: Sustainable Architecture

As the world faced environmental challenges, architecture evolved to meet the needs of sustainability. Green buildings, designed to minimize environmental impact, became the new standard. This shift was not just about technology; it reflected a growing recognition of humanity's responsibility to the earth. Ancient myths of harmony with nature, such as the Native American reverence for the land, found new expression in sustainable design. Architects and builders sought to create structures that honored the natural world, reinforcing the sacred connection between humanity and the environment.

The principles of sustainable architecture are rooted in the idea of creating buildings that are in harmony with their surroundings. This involves using renewable materials, incorporating energy-efficient technologies, and designing spaces that promote natural ventilation and daylight. The concept of biophilic design, which emphasizes the integration of natural elements into the built environment, draws inspiration from ancient practices and myths that celebrate the connection between humans and nature. Green roofs, living walls, and natural landscaping are examples of how modern architecture can create a more sustainable and harmonious relationship with the environment.

One of the key challenges of sustainable architecture is balancing the needs of human habitation with the preservation of natural ecosystems. This requires a holistic approach that considers the entire life cycle of a building, from construction to demolition. The use of sustainable materials, such as recycled and locally sourced products, helps to reduce the environmental impact of construction. Additionally, the design of energy-efficient buildings, incorporating technologies such as solar panels and geothermal heating, reduces the reliance on fossil fuels and lowers greenhouse gas emissions.

The concept of the "ecological footprint" has become an important metric in sustainable design, measuring the impact of human activities on the environment. Architects and urban planners use this concept to create spaces that minimize resource consumption and promote sustainable living. The development of eco-cities and green communities, which prioritize walkability, public transportation, and green spaces, reflects a growing recognition of the need to create more sustainable and resilient urban environments.

As we face the challenges of climate change and environmental degradation, sustainable architecture offers a path forward that honors the ancient wisdom of living in harmony with nature. By integrating modern technologies with timeless principles of design, we can create buildings and communities that are not only functional and beautiful but also sustainable and respectful of the natural world. The sacred scaffold that connects humanity to the environment continues to evolve, offering hope for a more sustainable and harmonious future.

10

Chapter 10: The Digital Age and Virtual Realities

The advent of the digital age brought about a new frontier of architectural innovation. Virtual reality and augmented reality allowed for the creation of spaces that transcended physical limitations. These digital environments opened up new possibilities for storytelling, education, and healing. Ancient myths found new life in these virtual realms, as creators drew on timeless stories to design immersive experiences. The digital scaffold became a bridge between the past and the future, blending myth, medicine, and architecture in unprecedented ways.

Virtual reality (VR) technology has revolutionized the way we experience and interact with architectural spaces. By creating immersive digital environments, VR allows architects to visualize and experiment with designs before they are built. This technology also offers new opportunities for education and training, enabling students and professionals to explore complex architectural concepts in a hands-on, interactive manner. Moreover, VR has the potential to transform healthcare by providing therapeutic environments for patients, such as virtual nature walks for stress relief or simulations for physical rehabilitation.

Augmented reality (AR), which overlays digital information onto the physical world, has also had a significant impact on architecture and construction. AR applications enable architects and builders to visualize and modify designs in real-time, streamlining the construction process and reducing errors. This technology also enhances the experience of existing architectural spaces by providing additional layers of information and interactivity. For example, visitors to historical sites can use AR to view reconstructions of ancient structures, gaining a deeper understanding of their history and significance.

The integration of digital technologies with traditional architectural practices has led to the emergence of innovative design approaches. Parametric design, which uses algorithms to generate complex and adaptive structures, is one such approach that has gained prominence in recent years. This method allows architects to create highly customized and efficient designs that respond to specific environmental and functional requirements. The use of digital fabrication techniques, such as 3D printing, further expands the possibilities for creating intricate and sustainable architectural forms.

As we continue to explore the potential of digital technologies, the boundaries between the physical and virtual worlds will increasingly blur. The architectural innovations of the digital age offer new ways to engage with space, culture, and history, while also addressing contemporary challenges in sustainability and healthcare. By embracing these advancements, we can build a future that honors the legacy of the sacred scaffold and continues to push the boundaries of human creativity and ingenuity.

11

Chapter 11: Rediscovering Ancient Wisdom

In the modern world, there is a growing interest in rediscovering the wisdom of ancient cultures. Traditional medicine, once dismissed as primitive, is now being studied for its holistic approach to health. Architectural principles from the past, such as biophilic design, are being reintroduced to create spaces that promote well-being. This resurgence of interest in ancient knowledge reflects a recognition that the sacred scaffold, built by our ancestors, still holds valuable lessons for us today. By integrating this wisdom with modern innovations, we can create a more harmonious and sustainable future.

Traditional medicine practices, such as Ayurveda and Traditional Chinese Medicine (TCM), emphasize the balance between mind, body, and spirit. These holistic approaches to health are gaining renewed interest as people seek alternatives to conventional medicine. Herbal remedies, acupuncture, and other traditional therapies are being studied for their efficacy and potential benefits. This blending of ancient wisdom with modern scientific research is leading to a more comprehensive understanding of health and well-being.

In the realm of architecture, the principles of biophilic design are being embraced to create spaces that enhance human health and well-being. This design approach seeks to connect occupants with nature by incorporating natural elements, such as plants, water features, and natural light, into the built environment. Research has shown that biophilic design can reduce stress, improve cognitive function, and promote overall well-being. By drawing on ancient practices that celebrated the connection between humans and nature, architects are creating spaces that nurture both the body and the spirit.

The revival of ancient wisdom is also evident in the growing interest in sustainable living practices. Traditional agricultural techniques, such as permaculture and agroforestry, are being reintroduced to promote sustainable food production and land management. These methods emphasize the importance of working in harmony with natural ecosystems, rather than exploiting them. By combining traditional knowledge with modern technology, we can create more resilient and sustainable communities that respect and preserve the environment.

As we look to the future, the integration of ancient wisdom with contemporary innovations offers a path toward a more balanced and sustainable world. By honoring the lessons of the past and applying them to the challenges of the present, we can create a future that is both innovative and deeply connected to the sacred stories that have guided humanity for millennia. The sacred scaffold that supports our journey through myth, medicine, and architecture continues to evolve, offering hope and inspiration for generations to come.

12

Chapter 12: Building the Future

As we look to the future, the journey through myth, medicine, and architectural innovation continues. The challenges we face, from climate change to pandemics, require new solutions that are informed by both ancient wisdom and modern science. The sacred scaffold, built on the foundations of myth and medicine, continues to evolve. Architects, doctors, and storytellers will play a crucial role in shaping this future. By honoring the past and embracing the possibilities of the present, we can build a world that is both innovative and deeply connected to the sacred stories that have guided humanity for millennia.

The future of architecture lies in the development of smart cities and sustainable urban environments. These cities will leverage advanced technologies, such as the Internet of Things (IoT), artificial intelligence, and renewable energy systems, to create efficient and resilient communities. By integrating these technologies with principles of sustainable design, architects and urban planners can create cities that prioritize the well-being of their inhabitants while minimizing their environmental impact. The concept of the "circular economy," which emphasizes the reuse and recycling of resources, will also play a key role in shaping the cities of the future.

In the field of medicine, the integration of digital technologies and personalized treatments will continue to revolutionize healthcare. Advances in genomics, telemedicine, and wearable health devices will enable more precise and effective treatments, tailored to individual patients' needs. The use of artificial intelligence and machine learning in medical research and diagnostics will accelerate the discovery of new therapies and improve the accuracy of diagnoses. By combining these innovations with a holistic approach to health, we can create a healthcare system that addresses the physical, mental, and emotional well-being of patients.

Storytelling will remain a powerful tool for shaping cultural narratives and fostering a sense of connection and understanding. As we navigate the complexities of the modern world, stories that draw on ancient myths and cultural traditions can provide valuable insights and guidance. These narratives can inspire resilience, foster empathy, and promote a sense of shared humanity. By preserving and reinterpreting the sacred stories of the past, we can build a future that is both rooted in tradition and open to new possibilities.

The journey through myth, medicine, and architectural innovation is far from over. As we face the challenges and opportunities of the 21st century, the sacred scaffold that has guided humanity for millennia will continue to evolve. By embracing both ancient wisdom and modern advancements, we can create a future that honors the legacy of the past while forging new paths of innovation and discovery. The sacred scaffold is a testament to the enduring power of human creativity and the timeless quest for knowledge, connection, and transcendence.

13

Chapter 13: The Power of Symbols

Symbols have been a fundamental part of human culture since the dawn of civilization. They convey complex ideas, beliefs, and emotions in a simple and universal language. From the ancient Egyptian ankh, symbolizing life, to the modern medical caduceus, symbols hold immense power in shaping our understanding of the world. These visual representations are often rooted in myth and have transcended time to influence various aspects of society, including medicine and architecture. The sacred scaffold of symbols continues to connect the past and present, enriching our cultural heritage.

The use of symbols in architecture can be traced back to ancient civilizations. The pyramids of Egypt, the ziggurats of Mesopotamia, and the temples of Greece were all imbued with symbolic meanings. These structures were designed to reflect the spiritual beliefs and values of their societies. In medieval Europe, cathedrals were adorned with intricate carvings and stained glass windows depicting biblical scenes and religious symbols. These visual narratives served as educational tools, conveying complex theological concepts to an illiterate population.

In medicine, symbols play a crucial role in communication and identity. The red cross, the rod of Asclepius, and the green cross are universally recognized symbols associated with healthcare and healing. These symbols convey trust, safety, and the promise of care. The use of symbols in medical practice dates back to ancient times when healers and physicians adopted specific emblems to signify their knowledge and authority. Today, these symbols continue to serve as powerful identifiers in the global healthcare landscape.

The enduring power of symbols lies in their ability to transcend language and cultural barriers. They serve as a bridge between different realms of human experience, connecting the tangible and intangible, the physical and spiritual. By understanding the historical and cultural significance of symbols, we can appreciate their role in shaping our collective consciousness. The sacred scaffold of symbols continues to evolve, reflecting the dynamic and interconnected nature of human society.

14

Chapter 14: The Healing Power of Nature

Nature has always been a source of inspiration, solace, and healing for humanity. Ancient myths and medical practices often emphasized the importance of living in harmony with the natural world. The concept of nature as a healer is deeply rooted in traditional medicine and has been validated by modern scientific research. The sacred scaffold that connects myth, medicine, and architecture finds a profound expression in the healing power of nature.

The practice of using natural elements for healing can be traced back to ancient civilizations. Herbal medicine, for example, has been used for thousands of years to treat various ailments. The use of plants and natural remedies is a common thread in traditional medical systems such as Ayurveda, Traditional Chinese Medicine, and Indigenous healing practices. These ancient traditions emphasize the holistic approach to health, recognizing the interconnectedness of mind, body, and spirit.

Modern research has further validated the healing properties of nature. Studies have shown that exposure to natural environments can reduce stress, improve mood, and enhance overall well-being. The concept of "forest bathing," or spending time in forests, has been scientifically proven to have numerous health benefits. This practice, rooted in Japanese culture, emphasizes the therapeutic effects of immersing oneself in nature. The incorporation of natural elements in healthcare settings, such as healing gardens and green spaces, has also been shown to promote recovery and enhance patient outcomes.

Architects and urban planners are increasingly recognizing the importance of integrating nature into the built environment. The principles of biophilic design, which emphasize the connection between humans and nature, are being applied to create spaces that promote health and well-being. Green roofs, vertical gardens, and natural ventilation are examples of how architecture can harmonize with the natural world. By creating environments that celebrate and respect nature, we can build a future that supports both human and ecological health.

15

Chapter 15: The Global Exchange of Knowledge

Throughout history, the exchange of knowledge across cultures has been a driving force behind the advancement of medicine and architecture. The sacred scaffold that connects myth, medicine, and architectural innovation is enriched by the diverse contributions of different civilizations. The global exchange of knowledge has led to the development of new ideas, practices, and technologies that continue to shape our world.

The ancient Silk Road is a prime example of how knowledge and ideas were exchanged across vast distances. This network of trade routes connected the East and West, facilitating the exchange of goods, culture, and knowledge. Medical practices, architectural techniques, and mythological stories traveled along these routes, influencing societies in profound ways. The introduction of Chinese herbal medicine, Indian surgical techniques, and Persian architectural styles to other parts of the world demonstrates the power of cross-cultural exchange.

In the modern era, the exchange of knowledge has accelerated with advancements in communication and transportation. The globalization of medicine and architecture has led to the sharing of best practices, research findings, and innovative technologies. International collaboration in medical research has resulted in groundbreaking discoveries and the development of new treatments for diseases. Architectural conferences and publications provide platforms for sharing ideas and fostering creativity among professionals from different backgrounds.

The importance of preserving and respecting cultural diversity in the exchange of knowledge cannot be overstated. Each culture brings unique perspectives and wisdom that contribute to the collective understanding of humanity. By embracing the richness of diverse traditions and fostering inclusive collaboration, we can build a more equitable and innovative future. The sacred scaffold of knowledge continues to grow, connecting people and ideas across the globe.

Book Description:

"The Sacred Scaffold: A Journey Through Myth, Medicine, and Architectural Innovation" is an exploration of the profound connections between ancient myths, medical practices, and architectural marvels. Spanning 15 chapters, this book delves into the origins of myths, the role of healing in ancient societies, and the evolution of architectural design through the ages. From the sacred geometry of medieval cathedrals to the digital frontiers of virtual reality, the book examines how these three domains intersect and influence each other.

The journey begins with an exploration of the myths that shaped early civilizations, providing a sacred scaffold upon which cultural values and scientific understanding were built. It then delves into the intertwined history of medicine and religion, highlighting the contributions of ancient healers and the enduring legacy of their practices. The book also examines the symbolic and functional aspects of architectural innovations, from the ziggurats of Mesopotamia to the skyscrapers of the Industrial Revolution.

As the narrative progresses, the book explores the impact of modern advancements in medicine and architecture, emphasizing the importance of sustainable design and the healing power of nature. It also highlights the global exchange of knowledge and the role of symbols in shaping our collective consciousness. Throughout the book, readers will discover how the sacred scaffold that connects myth, medicine, and architecture continues to evolve, offering valuable insights for the future.

CHAPTER 15: THE GLOBAL EXCHANGE OF KNOWLEDGE

With rich storytelling and thoughtful analysis, "The Sacred Scaffold" invites readers to embark on a journey through history, exploring the timeless connections that have shaped human civilization. This book is a celebration of the ingenuity, creativity, and resilience of humanity, offering a deeper understanding of the forces that continue to influence our world.

www.ingramcontent.com/pod-product-compliance
Lightning Source LLC
LaVergne TN
LVHW010443070526
838199LV00066B/6175